Juicing for Cancer Recipes Book

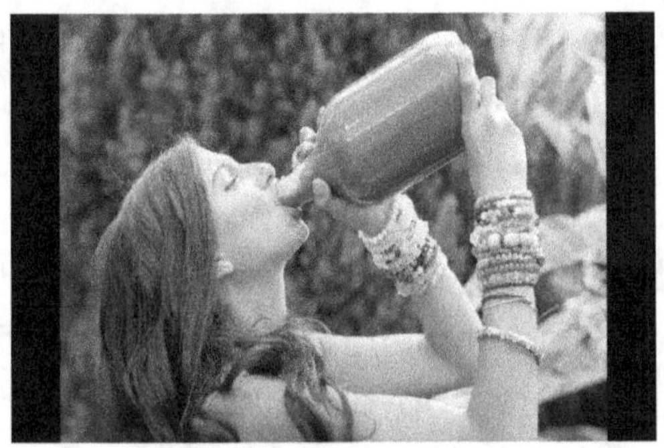

Natural and Healthy Delicious Meals for Healing and wellness

Isaac Hendricks

Table of Contents

Encouragement for readers to embrace a holistic approach to nutrition and well-being.

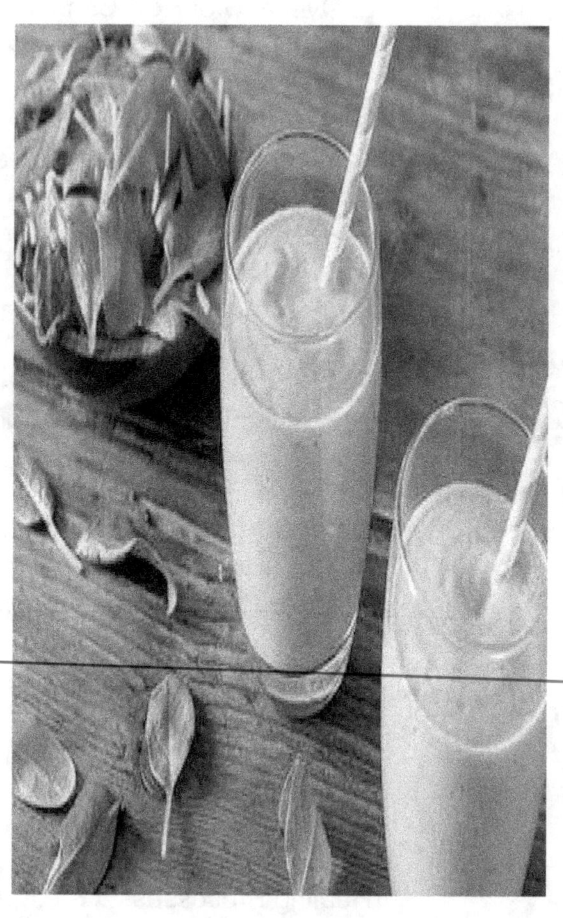

INTRODUCTION

Brief overview of the importance of nutrition during cancer treatment

In the face of cancer treatment, nutrition plays a pivotal role in supporting overall well-being and enhancing the body's resilience. A carefully tailored and nutrient-rich diet becomes an essential component of the patient's journey, influencing the tolerance to treatments, energy levels, and the body's ability to recover.

During cancer treatment, the body undergoes significant stress, and maintaining adequate nutrition becomes crucial to sustain strength and immune function. Proper nutrition can help manage side effects such as fatigue, nausea, and weight loss, ensuring that the body has the necessary resources to cope with the demands of therapy.

Key aspects of the importance of nutrition during cancer treatment include:

1. Immune Support: Nutrition plays a vital role in supporting the immune system, which is often compromised during cancer treatment. A well-balanced diet provides essential nutrients that contribute to the body's defence mechanisms.

2. Tissue Repair and Recovery: Cancer treatments can impact healthy cells along with cancerous ones. Nutrient-dense foods aid in cellular repair and recovery, helping the body cope with the effects of surgery, chemotherapy, or radiation.

3. Energy Maintenance: Cancer and its treatments can lead to fatigue, making it challenging for individuals to maintain energy levels. Proper nutrition, including a balance of carbohydrates, proteins, and fats, is instrumental in sustaining energy throughout the treatment process.

4. Side Effect Management: Certain nutrients and dietary choices can help alleviate common side effects of cancer treatment, such as nausea, loss of appetite, and changes in taste perception.

5. Optimising Treatment Effectiveness: Well-nourished individuals may better tolerate and respond to cancer therapies, potentially enhancing the effectiveness of treatments and improving the overall outcome.

In essence, the importance of nutrition during cancer treatment extends beyond mere sustenance; it becomes a critical component of holistic care, aiming to enhance the patient's quality of life and improve their ability to combat the challenges posed by cancer and its treatment modalities.

Introduction to the healing potential of juicing

In the realm of holistic health and wellness, the art of juicing emerges as a powerful ally, offering a natural and nutrient-packed approach to support the body's healing journey. As we explore the pages of this book, "Juicing for Cancer Recipes Book," we embark on a voyage into the world of juicing and its profound potential to complement and enhance the healing process, especially for those confronting the challenges of cancer.

Juicing, the art of extracting the essence of fruits, vegetables, and herbs into a liquid elixir, goes beyond being a mere beverage; it becomes a concentrated source of essential nutrients, antioxidants, and phytochemicals. These elements, harnessed in their purest form, offer the body a flood of bioavailable goodness, easily assimilated and readily absorbed.

Amidst the complexities of cancer treatment, where the body often undergoes rigorous challenges, juicing stands as a beacon of nourishment. It addresses the unique nutritional needs of individuals on this journey, providing a delicious and accessible means to fortify the body with vitamins, minerals, and healing compounds.

In the chapters that follow, we will delve into the science behind juicing, uncovering the specific ingredients renowned for their cancer-fighting properties. From morning boosters to evening healing elixirs, each recipe is crafted with intention, aiming to cater to the diverse needs and taste preferences of individuals navigating through cancer treatments.

Join us on this exploration of not just recipes, but of empowerment through knowledge. Learn how juicing can be a vital component of a holistic approach to well-being, complementing conventional medical treatments with the goodness that nature provides. As we sip through these pages, let us embrace the healing potential of juicing and embark on a journey towards wellness, one revitalising sip at a time.

CHAPTER ONE

Understanding Cancer and Nutrition

Overview of how cancer affects the body

Cancer, a complex and multifaceted group of diseases, manifests when the body's cells undergo uncontrolled growth and division. This abnormal proliferation forms a mass of tissue known as a tumour, which can interfere with normal bodily functions. Understanding how cancer affects the body is essential for comprehending the challenges individuals face during diagnosis, treatment, and recovery.

1. Unregulated Cell Growth:

   - Cancer begins at the cellular level, with mutations in the DNA leading to uncontrolled cell growth.
   - These abnormal cells form a mass or tumour, which may be benign (non-cancerous) or malignant (cancerous).

2. Invasion and Metastasis:

   - Malignant tumours have the ability to invade nearby tissues and organs, compromising their normal functions.

- Cancer cells can also enter the bloodstream or lymphatic system, spreading to other parts of the body in a process known as metastasis.

3. Disruption of Normal Cellular Function:

- Cancer cells compete with healthy cells for nutrients and space, disrupting the normal functioning of organs and tissues.
- This interference can lead to a variety of symptoms, depending on the affected organ or system.

4. Impact on the Immune System:

- Cancer can weaken the immune system, making it less effective in recognizing and destroying abnormal cells.
- Some cancers may also evade detection by the immune system, allowing them to thrive and spread.

5. Energy Drain and Weight Loss:

- The rapid growth of cancer cells requires a substantial amount of energy, often leading to fatigue and unintentional weight loss in individuals with cancer.

6. Production of Harmful Substances:

- Certain types of cancer cells can produce substances that interfere with normal physiological processes, leading to additional complications.

   - Depending on the location and type of cancer, organ function may be compromised, resulting in symptoms specific to the affected organ.

Understanding the impact of cancer on the body is crucial for tailoring effective treatments. Various cancer treatments, such as surgery, chemotherapy, and radiation therapy, aim to target and eliminate cancer cells while minimising damage to healthy tissues. By unravelling the complexities of how cancer alters the body's natural processes, medical professionals can devise comprehensive strategies to combat this formidable adversary.

Nutrition's significance in cancer patients' care

Nutrition plays a pivotal role in supporting cancer patients throughout their journey, from diagnosis through treatment and recovery. A well-balanced and nourishing diet is essential for maintaining strength, managing side effects, and promoting overall well-being. Here are key aspects highlighting the crucial role of nutrition in the context of cancer care:

Maintaining Strength and Energy

- Cancer and its treatments, such as chemotherapy and radiation, can lead to fatigue and weakness.
- Adequate nutrition provides the energy necessary to cope with the physical demands of both the disease and its treatments.

Supporting Immune Function

- A well-nourished body is better equipped to maintain a robust immune system.
- Proper nutrition enhances the body's ability to fight infections and recover from the effects of cancer therapies.

Managing Treatment Side Effects

- Nutrient-rich foods can help manage common side effects of cancer treatments, including nausea, vomiting, and loss of appetite.
- Adequate hydration and specific dietary choices can alleviate discomfort and improve the overall quality of life during treatment.

Preventing Malnutrition

- Cancer can lead to weight loss and muscle wasting, contributing to malnutrition.
- Proper nutrition helps prevent malnutrition, ensuring that the body has the necessary resources for healing and recovery.

Enhancing Tolerance to Treatment

- Well-nourished individuals often tolerate cancer treatments better.
- Maintaining a healthy weight and nutritional status can contribute to the effectiveness of chemotherapy and other therapeutic interventions.

Facilitating Tissue Repair and Recovery

- Cancer treatments can impact healthy tissues, leading to the need for repair and recovery.
- Nutrient-dense foods aid in the healing process, promoting the restoration of tissues affected by surgery or radiation.

Individualised Nutritional Plans

- Each cancer patient may have unique nutritional needs based on their diagnosis, treatment plan, and overall health.
- Registered dietitians work with patients to create personalised nutritional plans that address specific challenges and support optimal health.

Promoting Overall Well-Being

- Proper nutrition contributes to the overall well-being of cancer patients, both physically and emotionally.
- Enjoying nourishing meals can bring comfort and a sense of normalcy during a challenging time.

In essence, the role of nutrition in cancer care extends beyond mere sustenance. It becomes an integral part of a comprehensive approach to treatment, focusing on the specific needs of each patient to enhance their resilience, improve treatment outcomes, and foster an improved quality of life during the cancer journey.

Importance of a balanced and nutrient-rich diet

Maintaining a balanced and nutrient-rich diet is essential for overall health and well-being, and it becomes particularly crucial in the context of cancer care. Here are key reasons highlighting the significance of embracing a balanced and nutrient-rich dietary approach:

1. Optimal Nutrient Intake:
   - A balanced diet ensures the intake of essential nutrients such as vitamins, minerals, proteins, fats, and carbohydrates.
   - These nutrients play a fundamental role in supporting various bodily functions, promoting growth, and maintaining health.

2. Energy for Daily Activities:
   - A nutrient-rich diet provides the energy required for everyday activities, including work, exercise, and other daily tasks.

- Adequate energy levels are vital for cancer patients to cope with the physical demands of both the disease and its treatments.

3. Supporting Immune Function:

- Nutrient-rich foods contribute to a strong and responsive immune system.
- A robust immune system is crucial for cancer patients, as it helps the body defend against infections and recover from the effects of treatments.

4. Maintaining Healthy Body Weight:

- A balanced diet helps individuals achieve and maintain a healthy body weight.
- Maintaining a healthy weight is essential for cancer patients to support overall health and optimise treatment outcomes.

5. Managing Treatment Side Effects:

- Nutrient-dense foods can help manage common side effects of cancer treatments, including nausea, vomiting, and loss of appetite.
- Certain nutrients contribute to tissue repair and recovery, minimising the impact of treatment-related side effects.

6. Preventing Malnutrition:

- A balanced and varied diet helps prevent malnutrition, a common concern for cancer patients.

- Malnutrition can compromise the body's ability to cope with the challenges of cancer and its treatments.

7. Promoting Digestive Health:
- A diet rich in fibre supports digestive health, helping to prevent constipation and other gastrointestinal issues often associated with cancer treatments.

8. Individualised Nutrition Plans:
- Each person's nutritional needs may vary based on factors such as cancer type, treatment plan, and overall health.
- Individualised nutrition plans, created in collaboration with healthcare professionals, can address specific requirements and challenges.

9. Enhancing Quality of Life:
- A nutrient-rich diet contributes to an improved quality of life for cancer patients.
- Enjoying flavorful and nourishing meals can positively impact emotional well-being and provide a sense of normalcy during a challenging time.

In the journey through cancer care, embracing a balanced and nutrient-rich diet serves as a foundational pillar for health optimization. It not only provides the body with the necessary tools for recovery but also empowers individuals to actively participate in their well-being, fostering a holistic approach to health during and after cancer treatment.

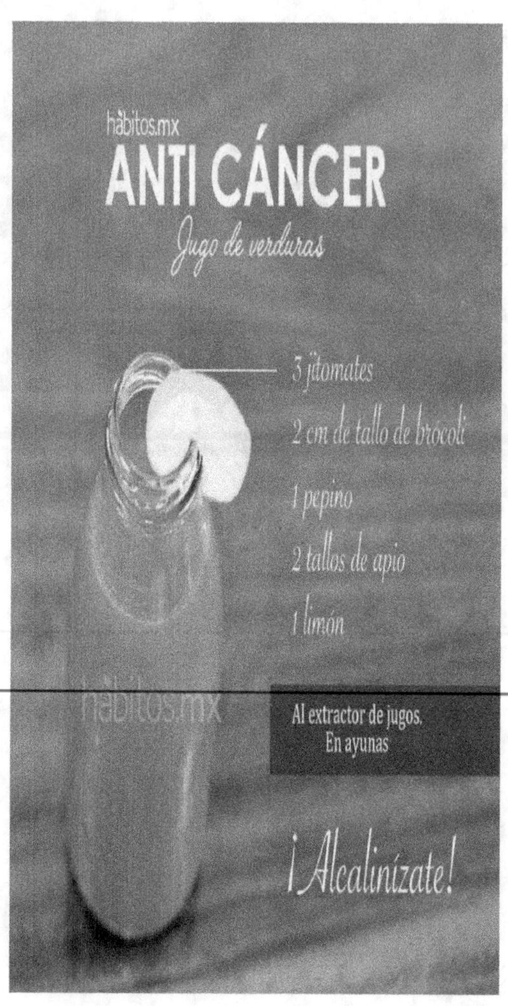
hábitos.mx
ANTI CÁNCER
Jugo de verduras
3 jitomates
2 cm de tallo de brócoli
1 pepino
2 tallos de apio
1 limón
Al extractor de jugos.
En ayunas
¡Alcalinízate!

CHAPTER TWO

Powerful Ingredients for Cancer Fighting Juices

Highlighting Fruits, Vegetables, and Herbs Known for Their Cancer-Fighting Properties

Nature has endowed us with a bounty of fruits, vegetables, and herbs that possess remarkable cancer-fighting properties. Incorporating these powerful ingredients into our diet can contribute to overall health and well-being. Here's a closer look at some of these nutritional superheroes:

- Berries:
 - Blueberries, strawberries, raspberries, and blackberries are rich in antioxidants, particularly anthocyanins, which have been associated with cancer prevention.
 - These berries also contain vitamins, fiber, and phytochemicals that support overall health.

- Cruciferous Vegetables:
 - Broccoli, cauliflower, Brussels sprouts, kale, and cabbage are members of the cruciferous vegetable family.

- These vegetables contain compounds like sulforaphane, known for their potential anti-cancer properties and ability to support detoxification processes.

- **Garlic:**
- Garlic is known for its organosulfur compounds, such as allicin, which exhibit anti-inflammatory and anti-cancer effects.
- Studies suggest that garlic may have protective effects against certain cancers, including those of the stomach and colorectal region.

- **Leafy Greens:**
- Leafy greens like Swiss chard, kale, and spinach are full of vitamins, minerals, and antioxidants.
- Their high fibre content supports digestion and may help lower the risk of certain cancers.

- **Turmeric:**
- The active ingredient in turmeric, curcumin, possesses strong antioxidant and anti-inflammatory qualities.
- Research suggests that turmeric may have potential in preventing and treating various types of cancer.

- **Tomatoes:**
- Tomatoes contain lycopene, a powerful antioxidant known for its potential to reduce the risk of certain cancers, especially prostate cancer.

- Cooking tomatoes enhances the bioavailability of lycopene.

- **Citrus Fruits:**
  - Oranges, grapefruits, lemons, and limes are rich in vitamin C, a potent antioxidant.
  - Vitamin C supports the immune system and may play a role in preventing certain cancers.

- **Green Tea:**
  - Green tea contains polyphenols, including catechins, which have antioxidant properties.
  - Some studies suggest that green tea may have protective effects against various cancers.

- **Ginger:**
  - Ginger contains bioactive compounds like gingerol with anti-inflammatory and antioxidant properties.
  - Research indicates that ginger may have potential in preventing and treating certain cancers.

- **Mushrooms:**
  - Certain mushrooms, such as shiitake and maitake, contain compounds like beta-glucans that may have anti-cancer effects.
  - Mushroom extracts are being studied for their potential in cancer treatment and prevention.

Incorporating a diverse array of these fruits, vegetables, and herbs into a balanced diet can contribute to a holistic approach to well-being.

While no single food can prevent or cure cancer, a combination of nutrient-rich foods provides the body with a spectrum of beneficial compounds that support health and may contribute to cancer prevention. Always consult with healthcare professionals for personalised dietary recommendations, especially in the context of cancer treatment.

Explanation of Key Nutrients and Antioxidants

Key nutrients and antioxidants are essential components of a healthy diet, playing crucial roles in maintaining overall well-being and supporting the body's various physiological functions. Understanding these vital elements is essential for crafting a balanced and nutrient-rich approach to nutrition. Here's an explanation of key nutrients and antioxidants:

1. Proteins:
   - Proteins are composed of amino acids, which are the building blocks of tissues, muscles, and organs.
   - Essential for cell repair, immune function, and the synthesis of enzymes and hormones.
   - Good sources include meat, poultry, fish, dairy products, beans, and legumes.

2. Carbohydrates:
   - Carbohydrates are the body's primary source of energy.
   - They are classified into simple carbohydrates (sugars) and complex carbohydrates (fibre and starches).
   - Good sources of complex carbs include whole grains, fruits, vegetables, and legumes.

3. Fats:
   - Fats are crucial for energy storage, cell structure, and the absorption of fat-soluble vitamins (A, D, E, K).
   - Healthy fats include monounsaturated and polyunsaturated fats found in olive oil, avocados, nuts, and fatty fish.

4. Vitamins:
   - Vitamins are organic substances that control the body's numerous metabolic functions.
   - Essential for immune function, energy production, and maintenance of skin, vision, and bone health.
   - Examples include vitamin C, vitamin D, vitamin A, and the B vitamins.

5. Minerals:
   - Minerals are inorganic elements necessary for the formation of bones, nerve function, and fluid balance.
   - Examples include calcium, iron, magnesium, zinc, and potassium.

- Found in dairy products, leafy greens, nuts, seeds, and lean meats.

6. Antioxidants:
   - Antioxidants are compounds that help neutralize harmful molecules called free radicals, which can damage cells.
   - Common antioxidants include vitamins C and E, beta-carotene, selenium, and various phytochemicals found in fruits and vegetables.
   - Berries, citrus fruits, nuts, and colorful vegetables are rich sources of antioxidants.

7. Fibre:
   - One kind of carbohydrate that the body does not completely digest is fiber.
   - Important for digestive health, regulating blood sugar levels, and lowering cholesterol.
   - Found in whole grains, fruits, vegetables, nuts, and seeds.

8. Omega-3 Fatty Acids:
   - Omega-3 fatty acids are essential fats with anti-inflammatory properties.
   - Essential for brain function, heart health, and inflammation reduction.
   - Found in fatty fish, flaxseeds, chia seeds, and walnuts.

9. Water:

- Water is essential for hydration, nutrient transport, temperature regulation, and overall bodily functions.
- Adequate hydration is vital for optimal health and well-being.

10. Phytochemicals:

- Phytochemicals are bioactive compounds found in plants that have potential health benefits.
- Examples include flavonoids, carotenoids, and glucosinolates found in fruits, vegetables, and herbs.
- These compounds may have antioxidant, anti-inflammatory, and anti-cancer properties.

In summary, a well-rounded diet that includes a variety of nutrient-dense foods ensures the intake of these key nutrients and antioxidants, promoting optimal health and supporting the body's ability to function effectively. It's important to maintain a balanced and diverse diet to provide the body with the full spectrum of essential nutrients for overall well-being.

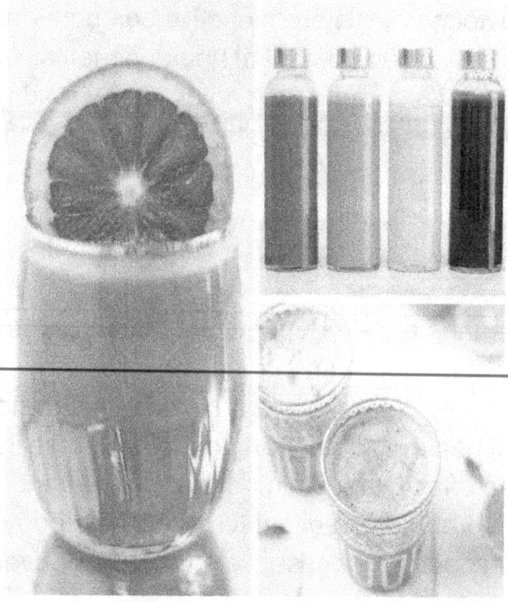
Healthy!
JUICING
RECIPES
supercharge your health!

CHAPTER THREE

Juicing Equipment and Techniques

Guide to Choosing the Right Juicer

Selecting the right juicer is a crucial step in making the most of your juicing experience. Different juicers have varying features and capabilities, catering to specific preferences and needs. Here's a guide to help you choose the right juicer for your lifestyle:

Juicer Types

- **Centrifugal Juicers:** Fast-spinning blades extract juice by shredding fruits and vegetables. These are quick and suitable for hard produce but may produce less yield and oxidise juice faster.
- **Masticating Juicers (Slow Juicers):** Crush and squeeze produce to extract juice slowly. Ideal for leafy greens and softer fruits, they yield juice with higher nutritional value and less oxidation.

Produce Compatibility

- Think about the kinds of fruits and veggies you want to juice. Centrifugal juicers are better for hard produce like apples and carrots, while masticating juicers excel with leafy greens, wheatgrass, and softer fruits.

Juice Yield

- Masticating juicers generally extract more juice from the same amount of produce compared to centrifugal juicers.
- If maximising juice yield is a priority, especially for costly or seasonal ingredients, a masticating juicer may be a better choice.

Nutrient Retention

- Masticating juicers operate at lower speeds, reducing heat and oxidation. This helps preserve more nutrients and enzymes in the juice.
- If retaining the maximum nutritional value of the juice is a priority, opt for a masticating juicer.

Ease of Cleaning

- Consider the ease of disassembly and cleaning. Centrifugal juicers typically have more parts and may be quicker to clean, while masticating juicers may have more intricate components.
- Dishwasher-safe parts and juicers with simplified designs can make the cleaning process more convenient.

Noise Level

- Centrifugal juicers tend to be noisier due to their high-speed operation, while masticating juicers operate more quietly.

- If noise is a concern, especially in shared living spaces, a masticating juicer might be a more suitable choice.

Juice Storage Time

- Juice from centrifugal juicers may oxidise faster due to the higher speed of extraction.
- If you prefer to make juice in batches for later consumption, a masticating juicer's slower extraction process may result in longer-lasting, fresher juice.

Budget Considerations

- Centrifugal juicers are generally more budget-friendly, while masticating juicers can be pricier.
- Consider your budget and how much you're willing to invest in a juicer based on your juicing preferences and frequency.

Additional Features

- Some juicers come with extra features like multiple speed settings, reverse functionality to prevent clogs, and attachments for making nut butter or sorbet.
- Assess these features based on your specific needs and preferences.

- Research juicer brands and read user reviews to gauge reliability, performance, and customer satisfaction.
- Choose a reputable brand with positive reviews to ensure a quality juicing experience.

Ultimately, the right juicer for you depends on your personal preferences, the types of produce you plan to juice, and your budget. Consider these factors carefully to make an informed decision that aligns with your juicing goals.

Tips on Juicing Methods for Optimal Nutrition

Achieving optimal nutrition through juicing involves selecting the right ingredients, using efficient methods, and maximising the benefits of each juice. Here are tips to help you get the most nutrition out of your juicing experience:

1. Choose a Variety of Produce:
- Include a diverse range of fruits and vegetables in your juices to ensure a broad spectrum of nutrients.
- Different colours signify varying phytonutrients, vitamins, and minerals, providing a more comprehensive nutritional profile.

2. Balance Sweet and Leafy Greens:
   - While fruits add sweetness and flavour, don't overlook the nutritional power of leafy greens like kale, spinach, or Swiss chard.
   - Aim for a balance to keep sugar content in check while boosting the nutrient density.

3. Rotate Ingredients:
   - Rotate your choice of ingredients regularly to introduce a variety of nutrients and prevent potential sensitivities or allergies from overconsumption of specific foods.

4. Juice Immediately or Store Properly:
   - Freshly juiced fruits and vegetables retain the highest nutritional value.
   - If you need to store juice, do so in an airtight, opaque container in the refrigerator, but try to consume it within 24 hours to minimise nutrient degradation.

5. Prep Ingredients Properly:
   - Wash and trim your produce thoroughly, removing any pesticides or contaminants.
   - Keep the skin on fruits and vegetables whenever possible, as it often contains valuable nutrients.

6. Alternate Ingredients for Better Consistency:
   - To enhance juice texture and consistency, alternate between softer and harder ingredients while juicing.

- This helps prevent clogs and ensures a smoother extraction process.

7. Use Citrus to Enhance Flavor:
- Citrus fruits like lemons and limes can add a burst of flavour to your juices.
- Their high vitamin C content also acts as a natural preservative and enhances the absorption of iron from leafy greens.

8. Include Herbs for Added Benefits:
- Experiment with herbs like mint, cilantro, or parsley for added flavour and potential health benefits.
- Herbs contribute antioxidants and phytonutrients to your juices.

9. Collect Pulp for Other Uses:
- Save the pulp generated during juicing for use in recipes such as soups, smoothies, or baked goods.
- This reduces waste and allows you to benefit from additional fibre.

10. Stay Hydrated Throughout the Day:
- While juicing adds valuable nutrients to your diet, it's essential to stay hydrated with water throughout the day.
- Water supports overall health and aids in the absorption of nutrients.

11. Experiment with Nutrient Boosters:
   - Consider adding nutrient boosters like chia seeds, flaxseeds, or wheatgrass to enhance the nutritional content of your juices.
   - These additions provide additional fibre, omega-3 fatty acids, and other essential nutrients.

12. Clean Your Juicer Thoroughly:
   - Regularly clean and maintain your juicer to prevent the buildup of residues and ensure optimal performance.
   - A clean juicer extracts juice more efficiently and maintains the freshness of the produce.

By incorporating these tips into your juicing routine, you can maximise the nutritional benefits of your juices and enjoy a flavorful and healthful experience. Remember that juicing should complement a balanced diet, and it's always advisable to consult with healthcare professionals, especially if you have specific health concerns or conditions.

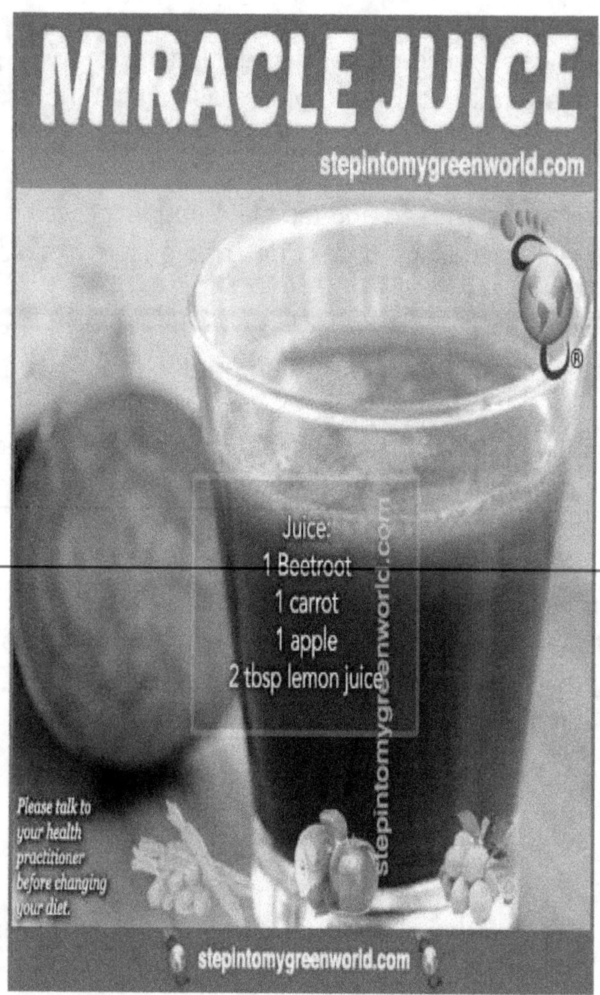

MIRACLE JUICE
stepintomygreenworld.com
Juice:
1 Beetroot
1 carrot
1 apple
2 tbsp lemon juice
Please talk to
your health
practitioner
before changing
your diet.
stepintomygreenworld.com
stepintomygreenworld.com

CHAPTER FOUR

Morning Boosters

Energising juice recipes suitable for the morning

Here are a couple of energising juice recipes suitable for the morning, designed to kickstart your day with a burst of freshness and vitality:

- Green Citrus Boost:
- **Ingredients:**
  - 1 cored and sliced green apple
  - 1 cucumber, peeled and sliced
  - 2 cups spinach leaves
  - 1/2 lemon, peeled
  - 1-inch piece of ginger, peeled
  - 1 cup water

- **Instructions:**
  1. Wash and prepare the ingredients.
  2. Juice the green apple, cucumber, spinach, lemon, and ginger.
  3. Dilute the juice with water and stir well.
  4. Pour over ice and enjoy this invigorating green citrus boost.

- Sunrise Energizer:

- **Ingredients:**
  - 2 oranges, peeled and segmented
  - 1 carrot, peeled and sliced
  - 1/2 pineapple, peeled and diced
  - 1-inch piece of turmeric, peeled
  - 1/2 cup coconut water

- **Instructions:**
  1. Wash and prepare the ingredients.
  2. Juice the oranges, carrot, pineapple, and turmeric.
  3. Combine the fresh juice with coconut water.
  4. Stir well and pour into a glass for a vibrant and refreshing sunrise energizer.

- Berry Burst Morning Delight:

- **Ingredients:**
  - 1 cup strawberries, hulled
  - 1/2 cup blueberries
  - 1/2 cup raspberries
  - 1 banana
  - 1 cup almond milk
  - 1 tablespoon chia seeds (optional)

- **Instructions:**
  1. Wash and prepare the berries and bananas.
  2. In a blender, combine the strawberries, blueberries, raspberries, banana, and almond milk.
  3. Blend until smooth.
  4. If desired, stir in chia seeds for an extra nutritional boost.

5. Pour into a glass and savour the berry burst morning delight.

These energising juice recipes are rich in vitamins, minerals, and antioxidants, providing a nutritious and refreshing start to your day. Adjust the ingredient quantities based on your taste preferences and enjoy the revitalising benefits of these morning juices.

Emphasis on boosting immunity and starting the day right

Certainly! Emphasising on boosting immunity and starting the day right is crucial for overall well-being. Here's a morning juice recipe designed to support immune health:

- Golden Immunity Elixir:

- Ingredients:
  - 1 medium orange, cut into segments and peeled
  - 1/2 lemon, peeled
  - 1-inch piece of ginger, peeled
  - 1 small carrot, peeled and sliced
  - 1/2 teaspoon turmeric powder or 1-inch fresh turmeric root, peeled
  - 1 tablespoon honey (optional)
  - 1 cup of coconut water or water

- Instructions:
  1. Wash and prepare the ingredients.

2. Juice the orange, lemon, ginger, carrot, and turmeric.

3. If using fresh turmeric, make sure to blend it thoroughly.

4. Mix in honey for added sweetness and potential immune-boosting benefits.

5. Dilute the juice with water or coconut water to your desired consistency.

6. Stir well and enjoy this golden elixir as part of your morning routine.

- Why This Juice?

- Citrus Fruits: Rich in vitamin C, known for its immune-boosting properties.

- Ginger: Contains anti-inflammatory and antioxidant compounds that may help support the immune system.

- Turmeric: Known for its anti-inflammatory and immune-modulating effects, thanks to curcumin.

- Carrot: Packed with beta-carotene, a precursor to vitamin A, which plays a vital role in immune function.

- Honey: Besides adding sweetness, honey has antimicrobial and antioxidant properties.

Starting your day with this Golden Immunity Elixir not only provides a refreshing and flavorful experience but also delivers a powerful combination of immune-supportive nutrients. Remember to adjust ingredient quantities based on your preferences and consult with healthcare professionals if you have specific health concerns.

CHAPTER FIVE

Afternoon Refreshers

Recipes for refreshing and hydrating juices to maintain energy levels throughout the day

Staying refreshed and hydrated is essential for maintaining energy levels throughout the day. Here are two refreshing and hydrating juice recipes to keep you energised:

- Cucumber Mint Cooler:

- Ingredients:
  - 1 peeled and sliced cucumber
  - Handful of fresh mint leaves
  - 1 lime, peeled
  - 1 cored and sliced green apple
  - 2 cups coconut water
  - Ice cubes

- Instructions:
  1. Wash and prepare the ingredients.
  2. Juice the cucumber, mint leaves, lime, and green apple.
  3. Combine the fresh juice with coconut water.
  4. Stir well and pour over ice.

5. Garnish with a mint sprig and enjoy this hydrating cucumber mint cooler.

- **Watermelon Citrus Splash:**
- **Ingredients:**
  - 2 cups fresh watermelon, diced
  - 1 orange, divided and peeled
  - 1/2 lemon, peeled
  - 1 cup coconut water or plain water
  - Fresh basil leaves for garnish

- **Instructions:**
  1. Wash and prepare the ingredients.
  2. Juice the watermelon, orange, and lemon.
  3. Combine the fresh juice with coconut water or plain water.
  4. Stir well and pour over ice.
  5. Garnish with fresh basil leaves for an extra burst of flavour.
  6. Enjoy this watermelon citrus splash for a refreshing and hydrating boost.

- **Why These Juices?**
- **Cucumber Mint Cooler:** Cucumber is hydrating, mint adds a refreshing element, and coconut water provides electrolytes for hydration.
- **Watermelon Citrus Splash:** Watermelon is high in water content, oranges contribute vitamin C, and coconut water enhances hydration.

These refreshing juices are not only hydrating but also packed with vitamins and minerals to help maintain energy levels throughout the day. Customise the recipes based on your taste preferences and enjoy these delicious and revitalising drinks.

Focus on combating fatigue

Combating fatigue is a common goal, and nutrition plays a crucial role in supporting energy levels. Here's a juice recipe focused on combating fatigue and providing a natural energy boost:

Energising Green Vitality Juice:

- **Ingredients:**
  - 2 cups spinach leaves
  - 1 cored and sliced green apple
  - 1 cucumber, peeled and sliced
  - 1/2 lemon, peeled
  - 1-inch piece of ginger, peeled
  - 1 kiwi, peeled and sliced
  - 1 tablespoon chia seeds (optional)
  - 1 cup coconut water or water

- **Instructions:**
  1. Wash and prepare the ingredients.
  2. Juice the spinach, green apple, cucumber, lemon, ginger, and kiwi.
  3. If desired, stir in chia seeds for an additional energy and nutrient boost.
  4. Combine the fresh juice with coconut water or water.

5. Stir well and pour over ice for a refreshing and energising green vitality juice.

Why This Juice?

- ☐ Spinach: Rich in iron, which is essential for preventing fatigue and supporting oxygen transport in the body.
- ☐ Green Apple: Provides natural sugars for a quick energy boost and contains antioxidants.
- ☐ Cucumber: Hydrating and contributes vitamins and minerals.
- ☐ Lemon: Adds a zesty flavour and vitamin C to support energy metabolism.
- ☐ Ginger: Known for its anti-inflammatory properties and potential to combat fatigue.
- ☐ Kiwi: Packed with vitamin C, potassium, and other nutrients for sustained energy.

This green vitality juice combines hydrating ingredients with nutrient-dense greens to combat fatigue and provide a natural energy boost. Adjust ingredient quantities based on your taste preferences, and incorporate this juice into your routine to support overall vitality. Remember to consult with healthcare professionals if you have specific health concerns or conditions related to fatigue.

CHAPTER SIX

Evening Healing Elixirs

Calming and nutrient-rich recipes for the evening

Here are two calming and nutrient-rich recipes for the evening to help you unwind and nourish your body:

Soothing Lavender Berry Bliss:

Ingredients:
  - 1 cup mixed berries (blueberries, raspberries, strawberries)
  - 1 banana
  - 1/2 cup Greek yoghourt (or plant-based alternative)
  - 1 tablespoon honey
  - A couple of fresh sprigs of lavender (for garnish)

Instructions:
  1. Wash and prepare the berries.
  2. In a blender, combine the mixed berries, banana, Greek yogurt, and honey.
  3. Blend until smooth and creamy.
  4. Pour into a glass, and garnish with fresh lavender sprigs.

5. Enjoy this soothing lavender berry bliss as a calming evening treat.

Golden Turmeric Chamomile Elixir:

Ingredients:
  - 1 cup chamomile tea, cooled
  - 1/2 teaspoon turmeric powder or 1-inch fresh turmeric root, peeled
  - 1/2 teaspoon cinnamon
  - 1 tablespoon honey
  - 1/2 teaspoon vanilla extract (optional)
  - Ice cubes

Instructions:
  1. Make chamomile tea and allow it to settle.
  2. In a glass, combine the cooled chamomile tea, turmeric, cinnamon, honey, and vanilla extract.
  3. Stir well until the ingredients are thoroughly mixed.
  4. Add ice cubes to the elixir and enjoy the calming and nutrient-rich benefits of this golden turmeric chamomile elixir.

Why These Recipes?

- Soothing Lavender Berry Bliss: Berries are rich in antioxidants, banana provide potassium and magnesium for relaxation, and lavender is known for its calming properties.
- Golden Turmeric Chamomile Elixir: Chamomile tea has calming effects, turmeric has anti-inflammatory properties,

and honey adds natural sweetness with potential soothing benefits.

These calming recipes incorporate nutrient-rich ingredients known for their relaxing properties. Enjoy them in the evening to unwind and promote a sense of tranquillity. Adapt ingredient amounts to suit your dietary requirements and tastes.

Supporting Relaxation and Aiding in the Body's Natural Healing Processes

Supporting relaxation and aiding in the body's natural healing processes involves incorporating calming ingredients that promote overall well-being. Here's a recipe with such ingredients:

Tranquil Lavender Mint Infusion:

Ingredients:
- 1 cup chamomile tea, cooled
- 1/2 teaspoon dried lavender buds
- 1 tablespoon fresh mint leaves
- 1 teaspoon honey (optional)
- Slices of lemon (for garnish)

Instructions:
1. Make a cup of chamomile tea and allow it to settle.

2. In a teapot or heat proof container, combine the cooled chamomile tea, dried lavender buds, and fresh mint leaves.

3. Allow the herbs to steep for about 5-7 minutes to infuse their flavours.

4. Strain the infusion to remove the lavender buds and mint leaves.

5. Add honey if desired, stirring until it dissolves.

6. Pour the lavender mint infusion into a cup and garnish with slices of lemon.

7. Sip slowly, allowing the calming aromas and soothing properties to promote relaxation.

Why This Infusion?

- ☐ Chamomile Tea: Known for its calming effects, chamomile may help reduce stress and improve sleep quality.
- ☐ Lavender: Contains compounds that may promote relaxation and alleviate stress.
- ☐ Mint: Adds a refreshing element and may contribute to easing digestive discomfort.
- ☐ Honey: Provides natural sweetness and may have potential soothing properties.

This tranquil lavender mint infusion is not only delightful in flavour but also incorporates ingredients known for their calming and healing properties. Enjoy it in the evening as a part of your routine to unwind, promote relaxation, and support the body's natural healing processes. Adjust ingredient quantities based on your preferences and consult with healthcare professionals if you have specific health concerns or conditions.

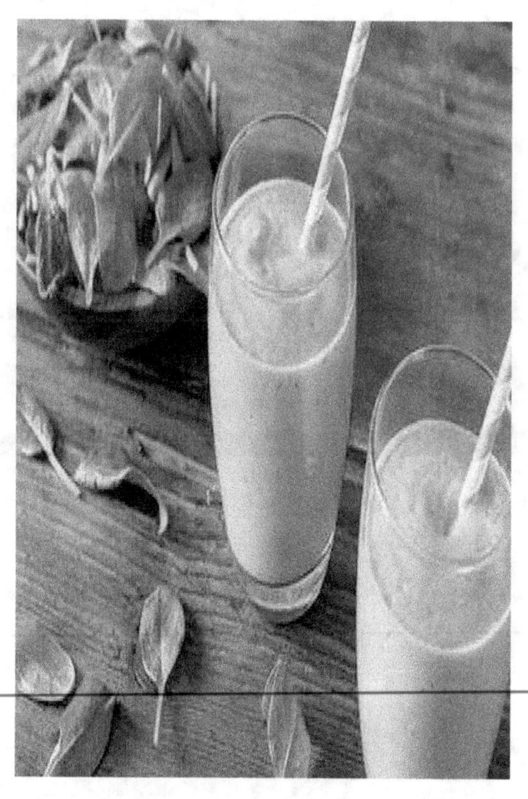

CHAPTER SEVEN

Tailoring Juices to Individual Needs

Guidance on adapting recipes to specific health conditions or personal preferences

Adapting recipes to specific health conditions or personal preferences is a thoughtful approach to ensure that the meals align with individual needs. Here is some guidance on how to modify recipes:

Consult with Healthcare Professionals:

- Before making significant changes to your diet, especially if you have specific health conditions, consult with healthcare professionals such as a doctor, registered dietitian, or nutritionist.
- They can provide personalised advice based on your health status and dietary requirements.

Consider Dietary Restrictions:

- Take note of any dietary restrictions, allergies, or intolerances. Common considerations include gluten-free, dairy-free, nut-free, or vegetarian/vegan preferences.

- Substitute ingredients accordingly, such as using gluten-free flour, plant-based milk, or alternative protein sources.

Adjust Portion Sizes:

- Modify portion sizes based on individual energy needs, weight management goals, or health conditions like diabetes.
- Consider using smaller or larger quantities of specific ingredients to meet calorie and nutritional requirements.

Modify Cooking Methods:

- Adapt cooking methods to suit specific health goals. For example, choose baking or grilling over frying for a lighter option.
- Use healthier oils or cooking sprays in place of butter or lard.

Choose Nutrient-Rich Ingredients:

- Focus on incorporating nutrient-dense ingredients to enhance the nutritional value of the meal.
- Include a variety of colourful fruits, vegetables, whole grains, and lean proteins to meet essential nutrient requirements.

Reduce Sodium and Sugar:

- Limit the use of salt and sugar in recipes, especially if you have conditions like hypertension or diabetes.
- Experiment with herbs, spices, and natural sweeteners to add flavour without compromising health goals.

Experiment with Alternative Ingredients:

- Explore alternative ingredients that align with dietary preferences or health conditions.
- For example, try using almond flour in place of wheat flour or using a plant-based substitute for animal products.

Control Portions and Mindful Eating:

- Watch your portion sizes to avoid overeating.
- Practise mindful eating by savouring each bite, chewing slowly, and being aware of hunger and fullness cues.

Record and Monitor:

- Keep a food diary to track dietary choices and monitor how specific foods affect your well-being.
- Adjust recipes based on your observations and consult with professionals if needed.

Educate Yourself:

- Stay informed about the nutritional content of various foods and their impact on health.

- Understanding the nutritional value of ingredients empowers you to make informed choices.

Remember that adapting recipes is a flexible and creative process. Be open to experimenting with different ingredients and methods to find what works best for your health and personal preferences. It's always advisable to seek professional guidance, especially when dealing with specific health conditions.

CHAPTER EIGHT

Incorporating Juicing into a Daily Routine

Practical tips on integrating juicing into daily life

Integrating juicing into daily life can be a rewarding and healthful addition. Here are practical tips to make juicing a sustainable and enjoyable part of your routine:

- Choose a Convenient Time:
- Select a time of day that fits well into your schedule. Many people find mornings convenient for a fresh start, while others prefer juicing as an afternoon pick-me-up.

- Prepare Ingredients in Advance:
- Wash, peel, and chop your fruits and vegetables in advance to save time when it's juicing time. Preparing ingredients ahead makes the process more efficient.

- Have a Variety of Ingredients:
- Keep a diverse range of fruits and vegetables on hand. This ensures you can create different

flavour combinations and benefit from a wide array
of nutrients.

- Experiment with Recipes:
 - Don't be afraid to try new combinations of fruits,
vegetables, and herbs. Experimenting keeps juicing
exciting and helps you discover your favourite
blends.

- Balance the Sweetness:
 - While fruits add sweetness, be mindful of their
sugar content. Balance sweet fruits with vegetables
like cucumber or celery for a nutrient-packed,
lower-sugar option.

- Consider Nutrient Boosters:
 - Enhance the nutritional content of your juices by
adding nutrient boosters like chia seeds, flaxseeds,
or wheatgrass.

- Batch Juicing:
 - Consider batch juicing for a day or two to save
time. Store extra juice in airtight containers in the
refrigerator, but consume it within 24-48 hours for
freshness.

- Invest in a Quality Juicer:
 - Choose a juicer that aligns with your needs.
Centrifugal juicers are quick, while masticating
juicers preserve more nutrients. Pick one that suits
your lifestyle.

- Clean Your Juicer Promptly:
- Clean your juicer immediately after use to prevent residues from drying and sticking. A clean juicer is more efficient and ensures better-tasting juice.

- Make Juicing a Ritual:
- Turn juicing into a ritual by creating a dedicated space in your kitchen. This helps establish a routine and makes it easier to stick to your juicing habit.

- Stay Hydrated:
- Although juicing contributes to hydration, remember to drink water throughout the day to meet your overall hydration needs.

- Listen to Your Body:
- Pay attention to how your body responds to different ingredients. Everyone's digestive system is unique, so adjust your recipes based on what works best for you.

- Educate Yourself:
- Learn about the nutritional benefits of various fruits and vegetables. Understanding the health benefits of your ingredients can enhance your commitment to juicing.

- Include Family and Friends:
- Make juicing a social activity by involving family or friends. Sharing recipes and experiences can

make the process more enjoyable and encourage consistency.

  • Celebrate Small Wins:
 - Acknowledge and celebrate the positive changes you experience, whether it's increased energy, better digestion, or improved skin health.

By incorporating these practical tips, you can seamlessly integrate juicing into your daily life, making it a sustainable and enjoyable part of your overall wellness routine.

Creating sustainable habits for long-term health

Creating sustainable habits for long-term health involves making gradual and lasting changes to your lifestyle. Here are practical tips to help you establish habits that contribute to long-term well-being:

  1. Start Small:
 - Begin with small, manageable changes. This makes it easier to incorporate new habits without feeling overwhelmed.

  2. Set Realistic Goals:
 - Establish achievable goals that align with your long-term vision for health. Break down larger goals into smaller, actionable steps.

3. Build Gradually:
   - Slowly build on your habits over time. Focus on one or two changes at a time to allow them to become ingrained in your daily routine.

4. Be Consistent:
   - Consistency is key to habit formation. Aim to practise your new habits regularly, even if it's in small increments.

5. Create a Routine:
   - Integrate your healthy habits into a daily or weekly routine. Having a set schedule makes it more likely that you'll stick to your commitments.

6. Find Enjoyable Activities:
   - Choose activities and exercises that you genuinely enjoy. This increases the likelihood that you'll continue them in the long run.

7. Involve Others:
   - Share your health goals with friends or family members. Having a support system can provide motivation and accountability.

8. Celebrate Milestones:
   - Acknowledge and celebrate your achievements along the way. This positive reinforcement helps reinforce your commitment to long-term health.

9. Adapt to Change:

- Be flexible and adapt your habits as needed. Life circumstances may change, and your habits should be adaptable to different situations.

10. Prioritise Sleep:
- Establish a consistent sleep routine. Quality sleep is essential for overall health and well-being.

11. Hydrate Regularly:
- Make drinking water a daily habit. Staying hydrated supports various bodily functions and can contribute to improved energy levels.

12. Practise Mindful Eating:
- Pay attention to your eating habits and practise mindful eating. Focus on nourishing your body with balanced and wholesome foods.

13. Incorporate Physical Activity:
- Find enjoyable forms of exercise and make them a regular part of your routine. This could include walking, cycling, swimming, or any activity you love.

14. Reduce Stress:
- Incorporate stress management techniques such as meditation, deep breathing, or yoga into your routine to support mental and emotional well-being.

15. Monitor Progress:

- Keep track of your progress. Whether through a journal, app, or other means, monitoring your journey helps you stay on course and identify areas for improvement.

16. Educate Yourself:
- Stay informed about health and wellness. Knowing the benefits of your habits can provide additional motivation.

17. Seek Professional Guidance:
- Consult with healthcare professionals or specialists for personalised advice tailored to your specific health needs.

18. Stay Positive:
- Cultivate a positive mindset. Focus on the benefits of your habits rather than fixating on challenges.

Remember that establishing long-term habits is a journey, and it's okay to make adjustments along the way. By gradually incorporating these tips into your daily life, you'll be better equipped to create sustainable habits that contribute to your overall health and well-being.

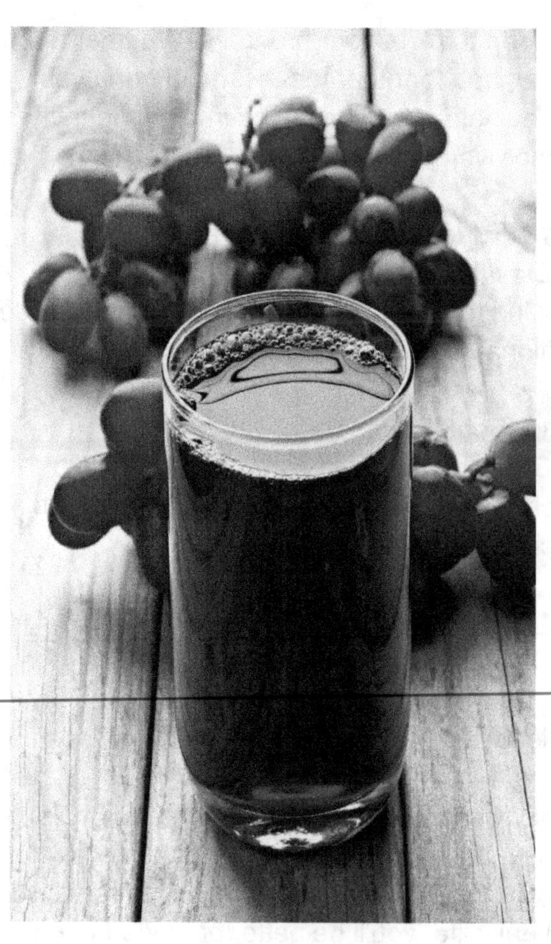

CHAPTER NINE

Success Stories and Testimonials

Real-life accounts of individuals who have benefited from juicing during cancer treatment

While there are anecdotal accounts of individuals experiencing benefits from juicing during cancer treatment, it's important to note that scientific evidence on the effectiveness of juicing as a standalone treatment for cancer is limited. However, some cancer patients have incorporated juicing as part of their overall nutritional strategy. Here are some real-life examples:

1. Chris Wark:

   - Chris Wark is a cancer survivor who shared his journey in his book "Chris Beat Cancer." He was diagnosed with stage III colon cancer at the age of 26. As part of his holistic approach to healing, Wark adopted a plant-based diet, which included juicing. He emphasised the importance of nutrition, exercise, and mental and spiritual well-being in his recovery.

- Kris Carr, a wellness advocate and cancer survivor, was diagnosed with a rare and incurable form of liver cancer. She chronicled her experience in the documentary "Crazy Sexy Cancer." Carr adopted a plant-based diet, including fresh juices, to support her overall health. She has since become an advocate for healthy living and shares her insights on incorporating nutrition into cancer care.

These individuals emphasise the importance of a holistic approach to cancer treatment, which may include dietary changes, exercise, stress management, and traditional medical interventions. It's crucial for individuals facing cancer to consult with healthcare professionals to develop a comprehensive treatment plan tailored to their specific needs.

While some cancer patients find comfort and potential nutritional benefits in juicing, it's essential to approach it as a complementary aspect of their overall care and not as a substitute for conventional medical treatments. Each person's experience with cancer is unique, and what works for one individual may not necessarily be suitable for another. Always consult with healthcare professionals for personalised advice and guidance.

Inspiring stories to motivate readers

Here are a couple of inspiring stories related to incorporating juicing into a cancer journey that could motivate readers for a "Juicing for Cancer Recipes Book":

Susan's Journey to Wellness:

- Susan, diagnosed with breast cancer, embraced a holistic approach to her treatment. Alongside conventional therapies, she integrated nutrient-rich juices into her daily routine. Susan's commitment to nourishing her body with a variety of fruits and vegetables played a supportive role in her recovery, inspiring others to explore the benefits of juicing.

David's Renewed Vitality:

- David, facing the challenges of chemotherapy, discovered the potential benefits of juicing to combat fatigue and enhance his nutrient intake. Experimenting with different recipes, David found a renewed sense of vitality and well-being. His story encourages others undergoing cancer treatment to explore the healing potential of fresh, vibrant juices.

Linda's Nutrient-Rich Healing:

- Linda, diagnosed with colon cancer, incorporated juicing as a complement to her treatment plan. Through personalised recipes focusing on cancer-fighting ingredients, Linda experienced increased energy levels and a sense of empowerment in her healing journey. Her story highlights the importance of nutrition in supporting overall well-being during cancer treatment.

Michael's Daily Wellness Ritual:

- Michael, a cancer survivor, adopted juicing as a daily wellness ritual post-treatment. The antioxidants and vitamins in the juices became an essential part of his lifestyle, contributing to his ongoing health and resilience. Michael's commitment to sustaining a healthy routine post-cancer inspires others to prioritise their well-being.

Emily's Journey to Recovery:

- Emily, a young cancer survivor, discovered the benefits of juicing to support her body's recovery after treatment. Juicing became a flavorful and enjoyable way for Emily to replenish essential nutrients. Her story resonates with readers, emphasising the importance of nourishing the body with wholesome ingredients during the healing process.

These stories aim to showcase the diverse ways individuals have integrated juicing into their cancer journeys, emphasising the potential benefits of incorporating nutrient-rich recipes into a holistic approach to health. It's essential for readers to consult with healthcare professionals and personalise their approach based on their unique circumstances

CONCLUSION

Recap of key points covered in the book

Here's a recap of key points covered in the "Juicing for Cancer Recipes Book":

1. Introduction to the Healing Potential of Juicing:

- ☐ Explores how juicing can be a valuable addition to a cancer wellness plan, providing essential nutrients and supporting overall health during treatment.

2. Overview of How Cancer Affects the Body:

- ☐ Discusses the impact of cancer on the body, emphasising the importance of nutrition in helping the body cope with the challenges of treatment.

3. The Role of Nutrition in Supporting Cancer Patients:

- ☐ Highlights the crucial role of nutrition in enhancing resilience, managing side effects, and promoting overall well-being for individuals undergoing cancer treatment.

4. Importance of a Balanced and Nutrient-Rich Diet:

- ☐ Emphasises the significance of a well-balanced and nutrient-rich diet, showcasing how juicing can contribute to meeting nutritional needs during cancer care.

5. Highlighting Fruits, Vegetables, and Herbs with Cancer-Fighting Properties:

☐ Spotlights specific fruits, vegetables, and herbs known for their cancer-fighting properties, guiding readers in crafting recipes rich in beneficial compounds.

6. Explanation of Key Nutrients and Antioxidants:

☐ Explores essential nutrients and antioxidants found in fruits and vegetables, explaining their roles in supporting the body's natural defences and promoting healing.

7. Guide to Choosing the Right Juicer:

☐ Provides practical advice on selecting the right juicer, considering factors such as juicing method, ease of use, and maintenance.

8. Tips on Juicing Methods for Optimal Nutrition:

☐ Offers valuable tips on juicing methods to maximise nutritional content, including the importance of fresh produce selection and proper juicing techniques.

9. Energising Juice Recipes Suitable for the Morning:

☐ Presents energising juice recipes tailored for the morning, designed to kickstart the day with refreshing and nutrient-packed combinations.

10. Emphasis on Boosting Immunity and Starting the Day Right:

☐ Discusses the immune-boosting potential of specific juice recipes, encouraging readers to incorporate these into their morning routines for optimal well-being.

11. Recipes for Refreshing and Hydrating Juices:

☐ Shares recipes for refreshing and hydrating juices, providing options to maintain energy levels throughout the day while staying well-hydrated.

12. Supporting Relaxation and Aiding in the Body's Natural Healing Processes:

☐ Introduces calming and nutrient-rich juice recipes suitable for the evening, promoting relaxation and supporting the body's natural healing processes.

13. Practical Tips on Integrating Juicing into Daily Life:

☐ Offers practical advice on seamlessly incorporating juicing into daily routines, making it an enjoyable and sustainable habit.

14. Real-Life Accounts of Individuals Benefiting from Juicing During Cancer Treatment:

- ☐ Shares inspiring stories of individuals who found support and benefit from incorporating juicing as part of their cancer treatment journey.

This comprehensive guide aims to empower readers with knowledge, practical tips, and inspiring stories, encouraging them to explore the healing potential of juicing as a complementary aspect of their cancer wellness journey.

Encouragement for readers to embrace a holistic approach to nutrition and well-being

Encouraging readers to embrace a holistic approach to nutrition and well-being is crucial for fostering a comprehensive and sustainable path to health. Here's a message to inspire readers:

Dear Readers,

In the pages of "Juicing for Cancer Recipes Book," we've delved into the transformative potential of nourishing your body with vibrant, nutrient-rich juices. Yet, beyond the recipes, we want to underscore the significance of embracing a holistic approach to nutrition and well-being.

1. Your Body as a Whole:
   - Understand that your body is a complex, interconnected system. Every choice you make, from the foods you consume to your lifestyle habits, plays a role in your overall well-being.

2. Nourishment Beyond the Plate:
   - Holistic well-being extends beyond what's on your plate. Consider the impact of stress, sleep, physical activity, and mindfulness on your health. Strive for equilibrium in all aspects of your life.

3. Listen to Your Body:
   - Your body communicates its needs and responses. Pay attention to how different foods and lifestyle choices affect you. Trust your intuition and make adjustments that align with your body's signals.

4. Fuel Your Body with Positivity:
   - Choose foods that not only fuel your physical health but also contribute to positive mental and emotional states. A healthy mind and body work synergistically to support your overall wellness.

5. Sustainability and Consistency:

- Develop long-term behaviors that you can stick to. Consistency is key to reaping long-term benefits. Small, gradual changes often lead to lasting transformations.

6. Connect with Nature:

- Recognize the healing power of nature. Whether through the nutrients in fresh produce, the grounding effect of outdoor activities, or the tranquillity of a peaceful environment, nature plays a vital role in holistic well-being.

7. Seek Support:

- You are not traveling alone. Seek support from friends, family, and healthcare professionals. Share your goals, challenges, and triumphs. A supportive community enhances the holistic nature of your wellness journey.

8. Practice Self-Compassion:

- Be kind to yourself. Understand that well-being is a dynamic process, and setbacks are a natural part of the journey. Approach your health goals with self-compassion, acknowledging that progress is a continuous evolution.

9. The Power of Choice:

- Remember that each choice you make contributes to your well-being. Whether it's choosing nutrient-dense foods, engaging in physical activity, or cultivating positive thoughts, your choices shape your health trajectory.

10. Celebrate Your Progress:
  - Commemorate each and every step forward, no matter how tiny. Recognize and appreciate the positive changes you make. These victories, however modest, fuel your motivation and commitment to a holistic and healthy lifestyle.

As you navigate the path to well-being, envision your journey as a tapestry woven with diverse threads—nutrition, movement, mindfulness, and more—each playing a unique role in the masterpiece of your health. Embrace the holistic approach with open arms, and may your pursuit of well-being be filled with vitality, joy, and a profound connection to the wonderful tapestry of life.

To Your Holistic Health and Happiness!

The Author of "Juicing for Cancer Recipes Book"

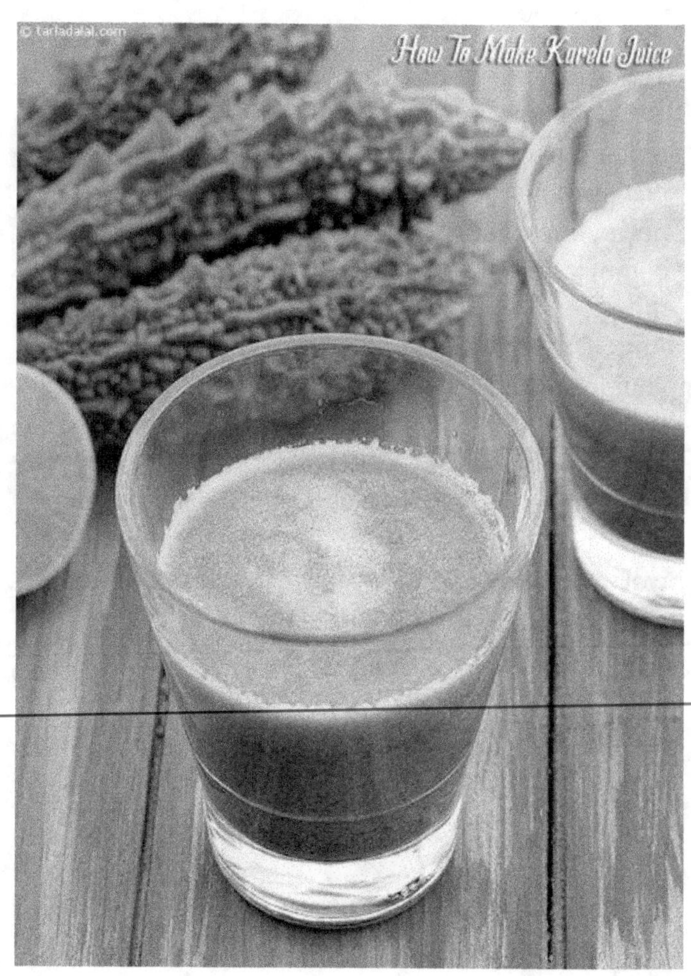
© tarladalal.com
How To Make Karela Juice